MEDITERRANEAN DIET COOKBOOK FOR TYPE-2 DIABETES

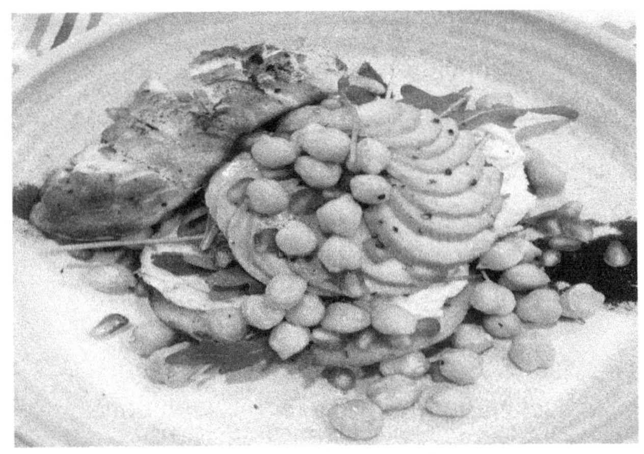

The Ultimate Guide With 50 Easy Recipes To Maintain Optimal Blood Sugar

Dr. Sylvia Roby

Table of Contents

Introduction

My childhood friend's grandmother Celestina, fought a tenacious enemy (Type 2 diabetes). Her golden years had been overshadowed by the illness, which made her feel disappointed and defeated. She had always served as the foundation of her family because she has been a true mother for everyone including me, so witnessing her suffering was agonizing. I went to a small supermarket to shop nearby, Just a few minutes from my friend's place. While doing some shopping for household items, I decided to gct a book for myself. Fortunately, I saw a Mediterranean Diet Cookbook created especially for those with Type 2 diabetes.

Without a doubt, I bought the cookbook because it will help my friend's granny live healthy and happy. I wanted to share my newfound optimism with her about how the Mediterranean diet may do wonders for controlling blood sugar. Celestina curiously opened the cookbook with her experienced eyes that had witnessed a lifetime of successes and difficulties. She went through its pages, her interest piqued and she was moved by the promise of a healthy lifestyle.

With unrelenting purpose, she dove into the cookbook. Her previously peaceful kitchen quickly became busy. She set off on a culinary adventure, preparing leafy green salads bursting with fresh vegetables, lean proteins seasoned with Mediterranean herbs, and Mediterranean breakfast bowls full of healthful grains and colorful fruits.

Weeks stretched into months as she continued to experiment with the recipes inspired by the Mediterranean, and then something extraordinary occurred. Her blood sugar levels started to level off. Her energy levels increased as she cut back on her prescription use. Her eyes were filled with relief and hope.

Her doctor, who had seen her problems for years, couldn't help but be amazed one day. Her overall health had substantially improved, and her blood sugar was now under control. Celestina, who had fought the enslaving grasp of diabetes with unflinching fortitude, celebrated her victory at that time. The cookbook provided her with more than just solace; it also gave her a fresh sense of direction. Celestine's health improvement has been Inspirational which made her family and friends amazed. She began talking about her experience with other older citizens, encouraging them to adopt the Mediterranean diet for the treatment of diabetes. Her kitchen evolved into a gathering place for fun, friendship, and delectable Mediterranean food.

What is Type 2 Diabetes?

In order to help your cells utilize glucose (sugar), your pancreas creates the hormone insulin. Pancreas produces the hormone insulin to aid your cells in using glucose (sugar). Your pancreas produces less insulin with time, and the cells start to reject it. Your blood starts to become too sugared as a result. Type 2 diabetes which include high blood sugar levels can cause heart disease, strokes, and even death. Diabetes Type 2 and type 1 are not the same. Those with type 1 diabetes have no insulin production from their pancreas. When you have type 2, your pancreas doesn't generate enough insulin and the insulin that it does create isn't always efficient. Both forms are subcategories of diabetes mellitus that result in hyperglycemia (high blood sugar).Despite being more common in adolescence, Type 2 diabetes primarily affects older people. Type 1 diabetes can occur at any age, however it commonly initially appears in children or young adults.

What causes type 2 diabetes to manifest?

Type 2 diabetes develops when the body's cells cease reacting to insulin and the pancreas produces less insulin than the body needs. They don't eat as much sugar as they should. Over time, your blood sugar levels rise. The failure of cells to react to insulin is known as insulin resistance. It is frequently caused by:

- lifestyle elements including obesity and inactivity
- Genetically flawed genes that prevent cells from operating correctly.

What symptoms and indications characterize type 2 diabetes?

Diabetes Type 2 symptoms often develop over time gradually. These include:

- Take hazy eyesight
- Fatigue
- Severe case of hunger or thirst
- Increased frequency of urine, usually during night.
- Healing from a cut or sore takes time.
- Your hands or feet may feel numb or tingly.
- Unjustified weight loss.

Side effects blood sugar levels cause?

The following are possible side effects of elevated blood sugar levels brought on by type 2 diabetes:

- Stomach issues, such as gastroparesis
- Eye issues, such as retinopathy brought on by diabetes
- Foot issues, such as ulcers on the legs and feet.
- Gum disease and other oral health issues
- Loss of hearing
- Heart conditions
- Renal illness
- Issues with the liver, such as nonalcoholic fatty liver disease
- Neural injury in the periphery.
- Abnormal sexual behavior.
- Skin ailments.
- Headache.
- Bladder infections as well as urinary tract infections.

How is diabetes type 2 diagnosed?

The blood tests listed below aid in the diagnosis of diabetes by your healthcare provider:

- Check your blood glucose level using the fasting plasma glucose test. It is preferable to take this exam in the morning at the workplace following an eight-hour fast (sips of water only during that time).
- The random plasma glucose test does not need a fast; it can be performed at any time.
- A1c, or glycosamino globulin hemoglobin testing, gauges your average blood sugar levels over a period of three months.
- A test for oral glucose tolerance measures your blood sugar levels both before and after consuming a sweet drink. The test assesses your body's glucose tolerance.

How is diabetes type 2 treated?

For Type 2 diabetes, there is no treatment. However, you may control the illness by leading a healthy lifestyle and, if necessary, by taking medicine. Collaborate with your medical professional to oversee your:

- Blood sugar: You can reach your blood sugar target with the use of a blood glucose meter or continuous glucose monitoring (CGM). In addition, your doctor could suggest routine A1c testing, insulin therapy, oral (pill) medicine, or injectable non-insulin diabetic drugs.

- Blood pressure: Maintain a balanced diet, quit smoking, and engage in regular exercise to lower your blood pressure. Beta blockers and ACE inhibitors are two types of blood pressure medications that your healthcare professional could suggest.
- Reduce your cholesterol by eating a diet reduced in sugar, salt, trans fats, and saturated fats. A class of medication called statins is one that your doctor could suggest to decrease cholesterol. With diabetes suggested by your healthcare professional. These oral medications can be used as tablets or in liquid form. For instance, the quantity of glucose your liver generates can be regulated with the use of a medication called metformin.

To improve the efficiency with which your body uses sugar, you can also take insulin. There are lot of insulin to be used at your reach

- You administer an injection of injectable insulin to yourself. The majority of people inject insulin into a bodily portion that is fleshy, like their abdomen. An insulin pen or a vial of injectable insulin are also available.
- You breathe in insulin by means of your mouth. Only a fast-acting version is offered.

Like a healthy pancreas, insulin pumps continually release insulin. Insulin is released into your body by pumps using a small cannula, which is a thin, flexible tube. By connecting a pump to a computerized device, you may control the amount and timing of insulin administered.

What kind of food should be in a Type 2 diabetic meal plan?

Meal planning for Type 2 diabetes should generally consist of:

Lean proteins: Seafood, eggs, and chicken are examples of proteins low in saturated fat. Tofu, beans, and nuts are examples of plant-based proteins.

Minimally processed carbohydrates: Refined carbohydrates, such as potatoes, spaghetti, and white bread, can quickly raise your blood sugar levels. Select carbohydrates such as whole grains like oatmeal, brown rice, and whole-grain pasta that raise blood sugar levels more gradually.

Less salt added: A diet high in sodium, or salt, can raise blood pressure. Avoid processed foods, such as those that are packaged or come in cans, to reduce your salt intake. Use healthy oils in place of salad dressing and select spices that are low in sodium.

No sugar added: Steer clear of sugary meals and beverages like soda, pies, and cakes. Drink either unsweetened tea or water.

Non-starchy vegetables: Due to their decreased carbohydrate content, these veggies don't raise blood sugar levels. Broccoli, carrots, and cauliflower are a few examples.

Benefits of the Mediterranean Diet for Diabetes

- Those who followed a Mediterranean diet high in nuts and olive oil had a far decreased chance of suffering a serious cardiovascular event like a heart attack or stroke. Also, these individuals had lower levels of central adiposity and other cardiovascular disease risk factors.

- The Mediterranean diet is a fantastic option for anybody trying to enhance their general metabolic health because of its emphasis on genuine, complete foods, especially those that are high in fiber.

- Research has demonstrated that the Mediterranean diet is superior to a low-fat diet when it comes to weight loss, and it also appears to lower the risk of chronic illnesses like metabolic syndrome and type 2 diabetes.

- Furthermore, the Mediterranean diet promotes social interaction and physical exercise in addition to being a diet. Therefore, regular meals with friends and exercise (even if it's simply walking) are also suggested.
- The body receives enough of vitamins from a Mediterranean diet: Vitamin deficiencies may be a concern for those with type 2 diabetes. It could cause an imbalance in the body's glucose levels. Vitamin C decreases blood glucose and improves insulin sensitivity. Diabetes is more likely to develop in those with low vitamin D levels. Furthermore, a vitamin deficiency leads to fluctuations in blood sugar and exacerbates diabetic symptoms.

Chapter 1: The Power of the Mediterranean Diet

The Mediterranean diet: what is it?

The main foods consumed in the Mediterranean Sea region, which includes Greece, Spain, and Southern Italy, make up the centuries-old Mediterranean diet. Though there are numerous similarities, this region does not have a single, consistent cuisine. Fish, red wine, whole grain breads, fruits, vegetables, rice, and pasta make up a large portion of the diets of these nations. In this area, red meat is rarely consumed. Herbs and spices are used in place of butter and salt. Food is rarely processed and is frequently prepared to a gentle texture.

Is it possible to manage Type 2 diabetes with a Mediterranean diet?

When picking a diet for someone with type 2, It is crucial to take into account how it will affect carbohydrate consumption and weight reduction.

There is proof that weight loss is possible with the Mediterranean diet.

Butter, processed meats, refined sugars, oils, and processed foods in general are minimal in Mediterranean diets. You'll see that regardless of the diet they follow, people with type 2 diabetes are recommended to limit or avoid all of these items. A lengthy list of items typical to a Mediterranean diet is provided below; there are plenty of delectable options to choose from. But take note: This diet also includes certain items that, if eaten carelessly, might cause weight gain. These consist of foods high in carbohydrates, such as rice, pasta, and potatoes. Thankfully, the Mediterranean diet comes in a variety of forms, and many of them do limit or eliminate high-carb items in favor of better options. For example, switching to brown rice or whole grain pasta can help reduce the quantity of carbohydrates ingested. Apart from its capacity to facilitate weight loss and lower carbohydrate consumption, the Mediterranean diet has demonstrated favorable effects on the progression of several chronic illnesses. Its most notable effect is that people who adhere to it have a lower risk of heart disease.

Mediterranean Diet Food Groups

Your diet need to revolve on these nutritious, raw Mediterranean foods:

Vegetables: Brussels sprouts, cucumbers, tomatoes, broccoli, kale, spinach, onions, and cauliflower.

Fruits: include melons, peaches, oranges, pears, strawberries, bananas, dates, figs, grapes, and strawberries.

Nuts and seeds: pumpkin, sunflower, and walnut seeds, as well as macadamia, hazelnut, and cashew nuts.

Legumes: Chickpeas, peanuts, pulses, beans, peas, lentils, etc.

Tubers: Yams, turnips, potatoes, sweet potatoes.

Whole grains: include whole wheat, whole-grain pasta, brown rice, rye, barley, corn, and buckwheat.

Seafood and fish: include shrimp, oysters, clams, crab, mussels, trout, tuna, mackerel, and sardines. poultry, such as chicken, duck, and turkey.

Eggs: duck, quail, and chicken.

Dairy: yogurt, cheese, Greek yogurt, and so on.

Herbs and spices: pepper, nutmeg, cinnamon, sage, rosemary, mint, garlic, and so on.

Healthy fats: Avocado oil, extra virgin olive oil, olives, and avocados.

Grocery Shopping Tips for Diabetics

<table>
<tr><td>

Meat & Fish.
- Chicken
- Turkey
- Oily Fish
- Tuna
- Salmon
- Mackerel
- Haddock
- Shellfish
- Shrimp/prawns
- Mussels

Oil
- Extra virgin olive oil

Condiments
- Hummus
- Tahini
- Balsamic vinegar

</td><td>

Dairy & Eggs
- Low-fat milk
- Low-fat yogurt
- Eggs
- Cheese
- Olive oil-infused margarine

Drinks
- Red wine

Bread & Grains
- Whole Grain bread
- Whole Grain pasta

Legumes
- White beans
- Black beans
- Chickpeas
- Red kidney beans
- Brown rice
- Buckwheat

</td></tr>
</table>

Nuts	*Produce*
● Seeds	● Onions
	● Garlic
	● Tomatoes
	● Aubergines/Egg plants
	● Courgettes/Zucc hinis
	● Mushrooms
	● Apples
	● Oranges
	● Pears
	● Bananas
	● Grapes

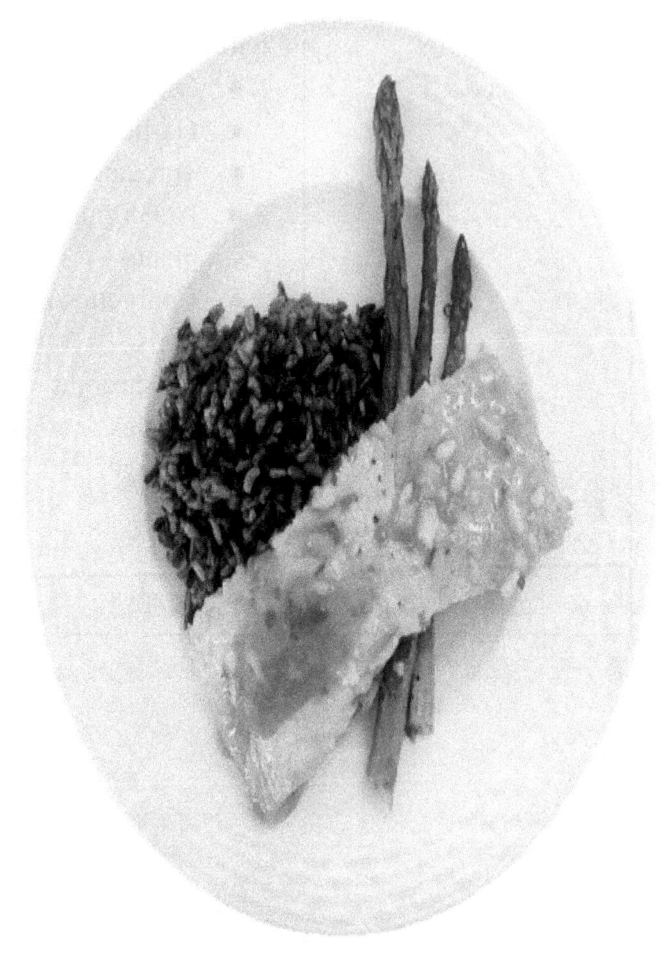

Chapter 2: Mediterranean Breakfast Recipes

Fast-cooking cereals

Ingredients:
One cup of low-fat milk or water
A dash of salt
1/4 cup of instant-cooking oats
One ounce of low-fat milk per person
One or two tsp honey, brown sugar, or cane sugar per serving
A dusting of cinnamon

Instructions:
1. In a small saucepan, mix the salt and water (or milk). Heat till boiling. After adding the oats, lower the heat to medium and simmer for one minute. After turning off the heat, cover and leave for two to three minutes.
2. Fill a 2-cup dish that can fit in the microwave with water (or milk), salt, and oats. Cook for one and a half to two minutes on high. Before serving, stir.
3. Garnish with your preferred mix of nuts, milk, sweetener, cinnamon, and dried fruits.

Southwest-Style Quesadilla

Ingredients:

Greaseless cooking spray

1/4 cup of thawed, chilled or frozen egg product

1/8 to 1/4 tsp salt-free combination of southwest chipotle spices

1 tortilla made with whole-wheat flour

Two tablespoons of part-skim mozzarella cheese, shredded

Two teaspoons of rinsed and drained canned black beans without added salt

Two tablespoons of chilled fresh pico de gallo or diced tomato, with additional for decoration

Instructions:

1. Apply nonstick cooking spray to a medium nonstick skillet. Heat a skillet to a medium temperature. Pour egg into a heated pan and top with spice mixture. Cook without stirring over medium heat until the egg starts to set around the edges and on the bottom. Lift and fold the partly cooked egg so that the uncooked piece flows underneath, using a spatula or big spoon. Cook the egg for a further 30 to 60 seconds over medium heat, or until it is cooked through but still glossy and juicy.

2. Spoon the fried egg onto one tortilla side right away. Add the two tablespoons of pico de gallo,

beans, and cheese on top. Gently press the tortilla to cover the contents.

3. Use a paper towel to clean the same skillet. Put some frying spray on the skillet. Heat a skillet to a medium temperature. Cook, flipping once, for about 2 minutes, or until the tortilla is browned and the filling is cooked through, while the filling is within the tortilla. Top with more pico de gallo if you'd like.

Egg Salad Toast with Avocado

Ingredients:
1/2 avocado
One-third cup celery
One-half tsp lemon juice
A smidgeon of spicy sauce
A dash of salt
One hard-boiled egg, chopped
One piece of whole-wheat bread
Instructions:
In a small bowl, mash avocado with celery, lemon juice, spicy sauce, and salt. Add hard-boiled egg and mix. Apply to toast.

Margarita Egg Pancake

Ingredients:

1/4 cup salsa tomatillo

One tablespoon of water

One big egg

One tablespoon of cotija cheese, crumbled

One tablespoon of freshly cut cilantro

Avocado, red onion or radishes cut thinly to serve

Instructions:

In a small pan over medium heat, bring salsa and water to a simmer. Create a little well in the center, then crack the egg into it. Cook for 3 to 5 minutes, covered, or until the egg is set. Take off the heat and sprinkle cheese and cilantro on top. If preferred, garnish with avocado, onion, and/or radishes.

Chickpea & Kale Toast

Ingredients:

One tablespoon of pure olive oil

Slicing 8 cups of kale

Two minced garlic cloves

One cup of rinsed canned chickpeas without additional salt

A dash of black pepper

Two toasted whole-grain pieces of bread

1/2 cup of feta cheese in crumbles

Instructions:

The oil should be hot through medium high heat in a big skillet . Cook the garlic and kale for approximately 4 minutes, stirring often, or until the kale is tender. Add salt, pepper, and chickpeas and stir. Divide the mixture equally among the bread slices. Add some feta on top.

Omelet with avocado and smoked salmon

Ingredients:
Two big eggs
One tsp of nonfat milk
A dash of salt
One teaspoon of extra virgin olive oil and half of a teaspoon, separated
1/4 sliced avocado
Single-oz smoked salmon
One tablespoon of freshly chopped basil
Instructions:

1. In a small bowl, beat eggs with milk and salt. In a small nonstick skillet, heat up 1 teaspoon of oil over medium heat.

2. Add the egg mixture and cook for one to two minutes, or until the bottom is set and the middle is still somewhat runny.

3. After flipping the omelet, heat for a further 30 seconds or until it sets. Move to a platter. Add salmon, avocado, and basil over top. Pour in the last of the 1/2 teaspoon oil.

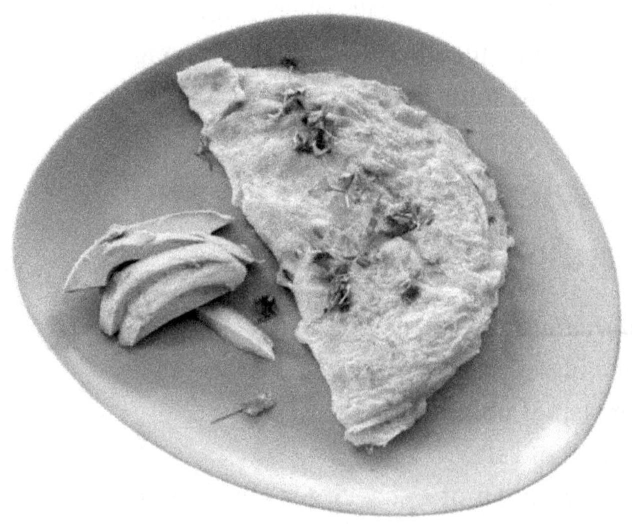

Chapter 3: Salad Recipes

Fattoush Salad

Ingredients:
2 loaves of pita bread
Superior quality olive oil
Halal salt
Split 2 tsp sumac; add more as necessary
One Romaine lettuce heart, chopped; one English cucumber, split in half; scrape the seeds; chop or slice into half-moon shapes.
Five Roma tomatoes, finely chopped; five green onions, chopped (both white and green sections); five radishes, chopped; remove stems; slice thinly.
Two cups of finely cut, fresh parsley leaves without stems
One cup of freshly chopped mint leaves (optional)

Vinaigrette or Outfit
1 lemon or 1 ½ limes, juiced
A quarter of a cup of pure olive oil
One or two teaspoons, optional, of pomegranate molasses
Add pepper and salt.
One tsp of sumac, one tsp of ground cinnamon, and tiny pinches of ground all spices

Instructions:

1. Bite-sized chunks of pita bread should be broken apart. Add the pita bread to a large skillet with 3 tablespoons of heated olive oil and heat until it shimmers. Fry for a little while, stirring often, until browned.

2. The cooked pita chips should be moved with a pair of tongs to a dish covered with paper towels so they can drain. Add sumac, pepper, and salt for seasoning.

3. Sliced radish, parsley, tomatoes, cucumber, lettuce, and green onions should all be combined in a big mixing basin.

4. In order to prepare the dressing, combine the lemon or lime juice, olive oil, salt, pepper, and spices in a small bowl, if using pomegranate molasses.

5. Lastly, incorporate the pita chips and more sumac, if preferred, and mix once more. Transfer to little plates or bowls for serving. Have fun!

Simple Broiled Asparagus

Ingredients:

1/2 pound of asparagus, with rough ends removed (baby asparagus is best if it's available)

Water

One lemon's zest

Instructions:

1. Bring 8 cups of water with 2 teaspoons of kosher salt to a boil in a big skillet or cooking pot.

2. Prepare a big dish of cold water next to it so that the blanched asparagus may have an ice bath in it. Once the water reaches a vigorous boil, include the ready asparagus.

3. Boil for 3 to 4 minutes (depending on thickness) or until tender. To halt the cooking process, remove with tongs, drain in a strainer, and then immediately transfer to a dish of cold water and let sit for one minute.

4. After draining, leave aside to cool somewhat (or refrigerate for a short while if serving as a salad). Arrange the asparagus on a serving plate and serve. Add pepper and salt for seasoning. Zest a lemon and sprinkle with quality extra virgin olive oil.

Use this Mediterranean salsa on top of your blanched asparagus, if you'd like.

Grilled Zucchini Salad

Ingredients:
4 sliced rounds of about 2 pounds of zucchini squash
1 teaspoon of organic ground cumin
1 lemon juice
1 minced garlic clove; Salt and pepper
1 cup of packed chopped fresh parsley
2 teaspoons of chopped fresh tarragon

Feta or goat cheese optional.

Instructions:

1. The zucchini should be put in a big basin. Sprinkle with cumin and drizzle with roughly 3 tablespoons of extra virgin olive oil. Using clean hands, toss to blend.

2. Add the zucchini on a hot grill or griddle in batches; do not overcrowd. Grill the zucchini for about 4 minutes, flipping them over a few times, until they are thoroughly cooked and have a beautiful char.

3. Return the cooked zucchini to the bowl. Add the lemon juice, salt, pepper, and fresh garlic for a sweet taste. To mix, toss. When adding new herbs, gently mix once more.

4. Spoon onto a serving tray, garnish with feta or goat cheese, if desired. Allow to come to room temperature.

Tomato Feta Salad

Ingredients:

6–7 medium-ripe tomatoes, cut into wedges (heirloom or on-the-vine tomatoes preferred)
1 medium red onion, halved and thinly sliced
3 minced garlic cloves
1/3 cup extra virgin olive oil
1 packed cup chopped fresh dill
1 packed cup chopped fresh parsley leaves

2 (½) teaspoons sumac, Kosher salt, black pepper

1 juiced lemon, 2 teaspoons white wine vinegar

Feta cheese, to taste

Instructions:

1. Gently toss the tomatoes, onions, garlic, parsley, and dill in a large salad or mixing dish.

2. After adding the sumac, taste and add salt and pepper as needed. Incorporate the extra virgin olive oil, white wine vinegar, and lemon juice. To mix, toss. To suit your tastes, add or subtract spice.

3. Move to a bowl or serving dish. Add a generous amount of fine feta cheese on top. Have fun!

Mustard Chickpea Salad

For clothing:

Half-tsp of Dijon mustard

One big lemon, squeezed and sliced

Half a cup of Greek extra virgin olive oil, either private Reserve or Early Harvest.

One minced clove of garlic

One tsp sumac

1/4 tsp coriander

1/2 teaspoon of cayenne

For the egg salad, add salt and pepper.

Two cans of rinsed and drained chickpeas

Two celery ribs, finely cut

Dice two Persian cucumbers (or one English cucumber with no seeds).

Two to three green onions, diced, both the green and the white portions
1/2 cup of red cabbage, shredded
Two chopped jalapeño peppers (optional)
1/2 cup of freshly cut parsley leaves, packed
1/2 cup of freshly chopped mint leaves, packed.
Five big sliced hard cooked eggs
Instructions:
1. Combine the dressing ingredients in a small dish or mason jar. For now, put aside.
2. Combine all the salad ingredients, excluding the eggs, in a large mixing bowl. Whisk the dressing briefly and drizzle it over the salad. Toss to blend.
3. Gently stir in the cut eggs one more time. Taste and adjust the pepper and salt. Garnish with more sumac. A few minutes should pass before serving.

Tabouli Bowl

Ingredients:
1/2 cup whole wheat bulgur.
Four firm Roma tomatoes, cut very coarsely
One English cucumber, often known as a hothouse cucumber, coarsely sliced
Two bunches of parsley, partially stemmed, well cleaned, let to dry, and finely chopped
Remove the stems from 12 to 15 fresh mint leaves, wash, pat dry, and cut very finely.

Four neatly sliced green onions, with white and green sections

Salted

3–4 tablespoons of lime juice (or, if preferred, lemon juice)

2-4 tablespoons Earlier Extra virgin olive oil harvest

Leaves of Romaine lettuce to serve, optional

Instructions:

1. After washing, soak the bulgur wheat in water for five to seven minutes. Make sure to thoroughly drain and press the bulgur wheat by hand to remove any remaining water. Put away.

2. As said previously, carefully cut the green onions, herbs, and veggies. Don't forget to put the tomatoes in a sieve to remove any extra liquid.

3. In a mixing basin or dish, combine the chopped veggies, herbs, and green onions. After adding the bulgur, salt it. Gently stir.

4. Add the olive oil and lime juice now, and stir one more.

5. Refrigerate the tabouli for half an hour after covering it for optimal effects. Move the mixture to a serving dish. Serve the tabouli with pita chips and romaine lettuce leaves, if desired. The leaves serve as "boats" or wrappers for the tabouli.

Mustard Potato Salad

Ingredients:

1(½) pounds of tiny potatoes, including red potatoes
Yukon gold potatoes, or new potatoes
Water
Teaspoon salt
One-cup chopped red onions
One-cup chopped fresh parsley
One-cup chopped dill, and two tablespoons capers
Dijon Vinaigrette:
cup of extra virgin olive oil
1/2 teaspoon Dijon mustard
1/2 tablespoon white wine vinegar
1/2 teaspoon crushed sumac
1/2 teaspoon black pepper
1/4 teaspoon ground coriander

Instructions:

1. After washing and scrubbing, pat potatoes dry well. A mandoline slicer may be used to finely slice potatoes.

2. Put the potatoes in a saucepan and cover with water for one inch. Heat till boiling, put some salt in.

3. Reduce the heat and boil the potatoes until they are soft, approximately 6 minutes or so (you should be able to pierce them with a fork).

4. In a small bowl, add the ingredients for the vinaigrette and whisk until thoroughly incorporated.

5. When cooked, remove from heat and make sure to drain properly. Transfer them to a large mixing bowl and drizzle with the Dijon mustard dressing right away. Toss gently to coat.

6. Add capers, onions, and fresh herbs, Gently toss to mix.

7. Place the potatoes onto a plate for serving. Before serving, give the potato salad some time to marinate for optimal results. It may be chilled for about an hour, but before serving, make careful to bring it to room temperature.

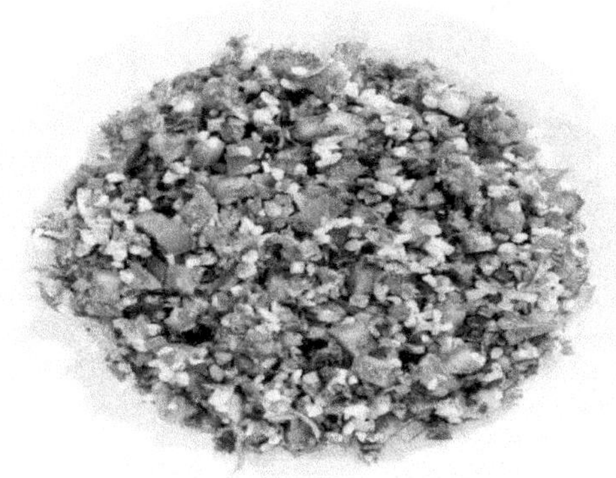

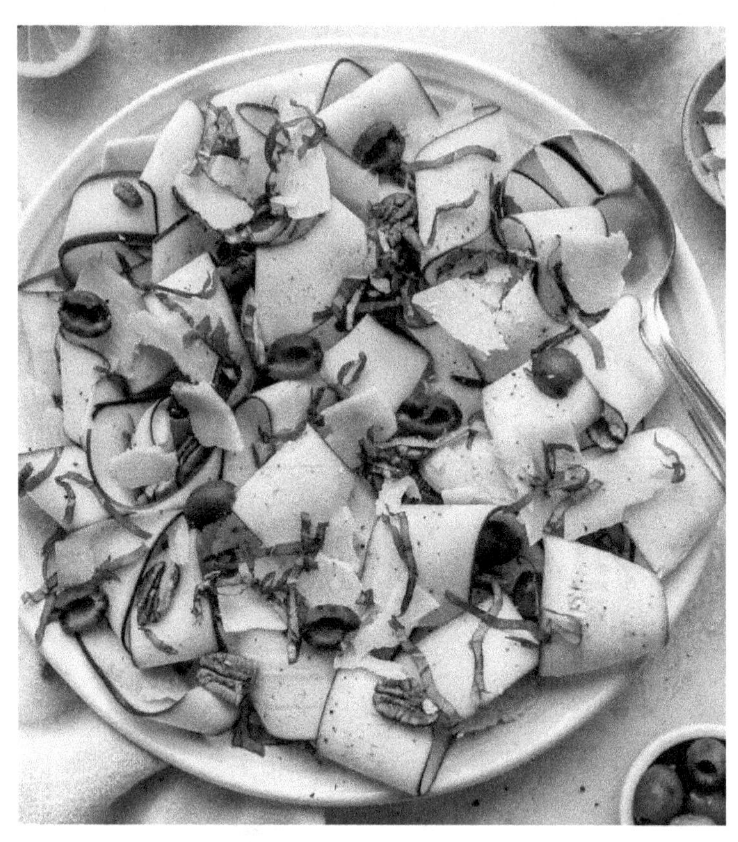

Chapter 4: Soup Recipes

Green Tomato Soup

Ingredients:

Two teaspoons of pure olive oil

1 cup of carrots, chopped

Sliced fennel (one cup); save fronds for garnish.

1/2 cup finely diced onion

Two tsp finely chopped garlic

1/4 teaspoon of coriander powder

Salt, ½ teaspoon

Six cups of vegetable broth low in salt

One fifteen-oz can of diced tomatoes with oregano, garlic, and basil that hasn't been salted

One small head (1 1/2 pounds) of chopped green cabbage

One fifteen-ounce can of washed and unsalted cannellini beans

Two tsp of sugar

One teaspoon of freshly chopped oregano

Zest of lemon for garnish

Instructions:

1. In a big, heavy saucepan, heat the oil over medium-high heat. Incorporate the carrots, fennel, and onion; stir-fry for approximately five minutes, or until the vegetables begin to soften.

2. Add the garlic, coriander, and salt; simmer for about a minute, stirring regularly, until aromatic.

3. Make sure the tomato and broth should be boiled. Adjust heat to medium after adding cabbage. Simmer for 20 to 25 minutes, stirring often, or until the cabbage is soft.

4. Add the beans, sugar, and oregano, and simmer for 3 minutes, or until the beans are well cooked.

5. Serve right away and garnish with saved fennel fronds and lemon zest, if preferred.

White Bean Soup with Shrimp and Tomato

Ingredients:
Three tablespoons pure olive oil
One pound of raw shrimp, peeled and deveined (26–30 per pound)
One tsp powdered ancho chili
Split a ½ teaspoon of salt.
Half a teaspoon of ground pepper, split
Diced one medium onion
Three minced garlic cloves
A tsp of finely ground red pepper
One 28-oz can of whole peeled tomatoes without additional salt
Two cups of chicken broth, unsalted

One 14-ounce can of white beans without additional salt

Two ounces of little whole-wheat pasta, such orzo

1/4 cup chopped, pitted Kalamata olives

Two teaspoons of chopped, rinsed, and

Freshly chopped parsley as a garnish

Instructions:

1. The oil should be heated in a big saucepan for very few minutes. Add the shrimp and season with 1/4 teaspoon each of salt and pepper and chili powder.

2. Cook for approximately 3 minutes, stirring now and again, or until just cooked through. Using a slotted spoon, transfer to a spotless plate.

3. To the pan, add the onion and the remaining 1/4 tsp of salt and pepper. Cook for 3 to 4 minutes, stirring often, or until transparent.

4. Add the crushed red pepper and garlic, and heat for approximately 30 seconds, or until fragrant. Make sure tomato and broth should be boiled. After adjusting the heat to a simmer, cook, covered, for ten minutes.

5. Using a potato masher, roughly mash the tomatoes, leaving some lumps. Add the beans, mashing some but leaving most whole. Bring back to a boil on high heat. Pasta should be added and cooked for 8 to 10 minutes, tossing often and cooking uncovered, until it is just soft.

6. Add the shrimp, capers, and olives and stir. If preferred, garnish the soup with parsley before serving.

Fish and Shrimp Stew

Ingredients:
Eight ounces of skinless sea bass or cod fillets
Six ounces of uncooked, peeled and deveined shrimp (31–40 per pound)
1/3 cup finely chopped onion
Two celery stalks, cut
1/2 tsp finely chopped garlic
Two tsp pure virgin olive oil
One cup chicken broth with reduced sodium
1/4 cup low-sodium chicken broth
One 14.5-oz can of drained diced tomatoes without additional salt
One eight-oz can of tomato sauce without additional salt
1 tsp crushed dried oregano
Salt, ¼ teaspoon
One-half teaspoon of ground black pepper
One tablespoon of freshly chopped parsley
Instructions:
1. Fish should be cut into 1 1/2-inch chunks. Slice the shrimp lengthwise in half. Store in the fridge until needed.

2. The oil should be heated in a big saucepan for very few minutes. Add the onion, celery, and garlic; simmer for approximately 5 minutes, stirring often, or until softened.

3. Stir in 1 cup broth and wine very carefully. Heat till boiling. After five minutes, lower the heat to a simmer.

4. Add the tomato sauce, oregano, salt, pepper, and drained tomatoes and stir. Bring the mixture back to a boil, lower the heat to a simmer, cover, and cook for five minutes.

5. Add shrimp and fish and stir gently. Bring back to a boil and turn down the heat right away. For three to five minutes, or until the shrimp become opaque, cover and boil the fish until it flake easily with a fork. Before serving, add a parsley sprinkle.

Pasta with Vegetables

Ingredients:
One tablespoon of pure olive oil
Two cups of frozen chopped and thawed bell pepper and onion mix
Two minced garlic cloves
1/4 teaspoon ground red pepper to give preferred taste
One 28-oz can of crushed tomatoes—ideally roasted over a fire

One fifteen-oz can of reduced-sodium chicken broth or veggie broth

1/2 cup boiling water

One tsp of dried marjoram or basil

One 6-to 9-ounce bag of frozen or fresh meat or cheese ravioli, ideally whole-wheat

Two cups chopped zucchini, or around two medium

Ground pepper freshly to taste

Instructions:

1. The oil should be heated in a big saucepan for very few minutes. Stir for one minute after adding the pepper-onion mixture, garlic, and crushed red pepper, if using.

2. Add the tomatoes, broth, water, and basil (or marjoram); increase the heat to high and bring to a rolling boil.

3. Cook the ravioli for three minutes shorter than instructed on the packaging. Return to a boil and add the zucchini. Simmer for 3 minutes or until the zucchini is crisp-tender. Use pepper to season.

Filling Spinach & Chickpea Stew

Ingredients:

Two fifteen-ounce cans of low-sodium chickpeas, washed and split

One tsp of olive oil

Turkey ground (93% lean) in 12 ounces

One-half teaspoon of dry oregano

1/2 teaspoon ground fennel seeds

A tsp of finely ground red pepper

1 cup of chopped medium onions

Diced two medium carrots (3/4 cup)

Half a teaspoon of garlic powder or four chopped garlic cloves

Three tsp tomato paste

One carton of low-sodium chicken broth (32 ounces; 4 cups)

A smidgeon of ground pepper

A tsp of salt

Three cups (8 oz.) of individually quick-frozen spinach

Optional: ¼ cup of grated Parmesan cheese

Instructions:

1. Use a fork or potato masher to mash one can of chickpeas. Put away.

2. The oil should be heated in a big saucepan for very few minutes. Add the crushed red pepper, fennel seeds, oregano, and turkey. Cook for two to three minutes, breaking up the turkey with a wooden spoon, or until it is no longer pink.

3. Add the garlic (or garlic powder), onion, and carrots. Simmer for 3 to 4 minutes, stirring often, or until aromatic and softened. Paste the tomato in. Stir and cook for 30 seconds.

4. Add salt, pepper, and whole and crushed chickpeas to the saucepan along with the stock. Put a lid on it and simmer it.

5. Lower the heat to low and quickly simmer the veggies, covered, for approximately 10 minutes, or until they are soft and the flavors have melded.

6. Put in the spinach and turn the heat up to medium-high. Stir and cook for 1 to 2 minutes, or until the spinach is well cooked. Spoon soup into individual dishes. If preferred, sprinkle 1 tablespoon of Parmesan cheese over each serving.

Mediterranean Diet Stew Made Slowly

Ingredients:

Two 14-oz cans of fire-roasted diced tomatoes without additional salt

3 cups of vegetable broth with minimal sodium

One cup of onion, diced coarsely

3/4 cup finely diced carrot

Four minced garlic cloves

One tsp of dehydrated oregano

A smidgeon of salt

A tsp of finely ground red pepper

A smidgeon of ground pepper

One fifteen-ounce can of washed and split, salt-free chickpeas

One bunch of stemmed and chopped lacinato kale (approximately 8 cups)

One-third cup lemon juice

Three tablespoons pure olive oil

Fresh basil leaves, ripped if they're big

Six slices of lemon (optional)

Instructions:

1. In a 4-quart slow cooker, combine tomatoes, broth, onion, carrot, garlic, oregano, salt, crushed red pepper, and pepper. Cook on Low for six hours with a cover on.

2. Pour 1/4 cup of the slow cooker's cooking liquid into a small basin. Add the two tablespoons of chickpeas and mash them well with a fork.

3. To the mixture in the slow cooker, add the mashed chickpeas, greens, lemon juice, and the remaining whole chickpeas. Mix well to blend. After the kale is soft, approximately 30 minutes, simmer it covered on Low.

4. Evenly portion the stew into six dishes and pour in some oil. Add basil as a garnish. If preferred, present with slices of lemon.

Filling Minestrone

Ingredients:

Two tsp extra virgin olive oil

Three medium leeks, thinly cut, cleaned (see Tip) and trimmed

Four cups of vegetarian or reduced-sodium chicken broth

1 cup of water

One big diced red potato

Two tspn of dried thyme

Salt, ¼ teaspoon

1/4 tsp finely ground pepper

One-half cup whole-wheat orzo

One 15-oz can of rinsed white beans

Two medium zucchini, finely cut after being quartered

One pound of freshly cut spinach without stems

Two tsp of apple vinegar

Two teaspoons of freshly grated Parmigiano-Reggiano parmesan cheese

Instructions:

1. In a big soup pot or Dutch oven, heat the oil over medium-high heat. Add the leeks and simmer for approximately 3 minutes, stirring now and again, until tender.

2. Add the potato, thyme, broth, water, salt, and pepper. After bringing to a boil, lower the heat, and simmer for five minutes with a lid on.

3. Add the orzo and simmer for 5 minutes, slightly covered and stirring now and again to avoid sticking. Cook the pasta and veggies for a further 8 minutes or until they are cooked, while partially covered, after adding the beans and zucchini.

4. Add the spinach and simmer, stirring, for 2 minutes or until wilted. Use some vinegar to season the soup. Spoon into dishes and sprinkle with Parmesan cheese.

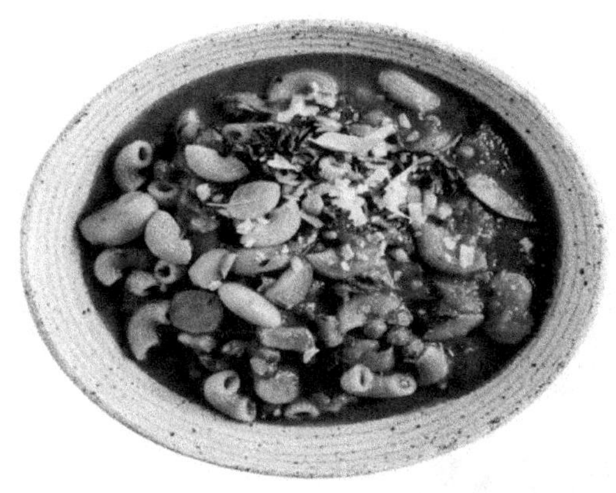

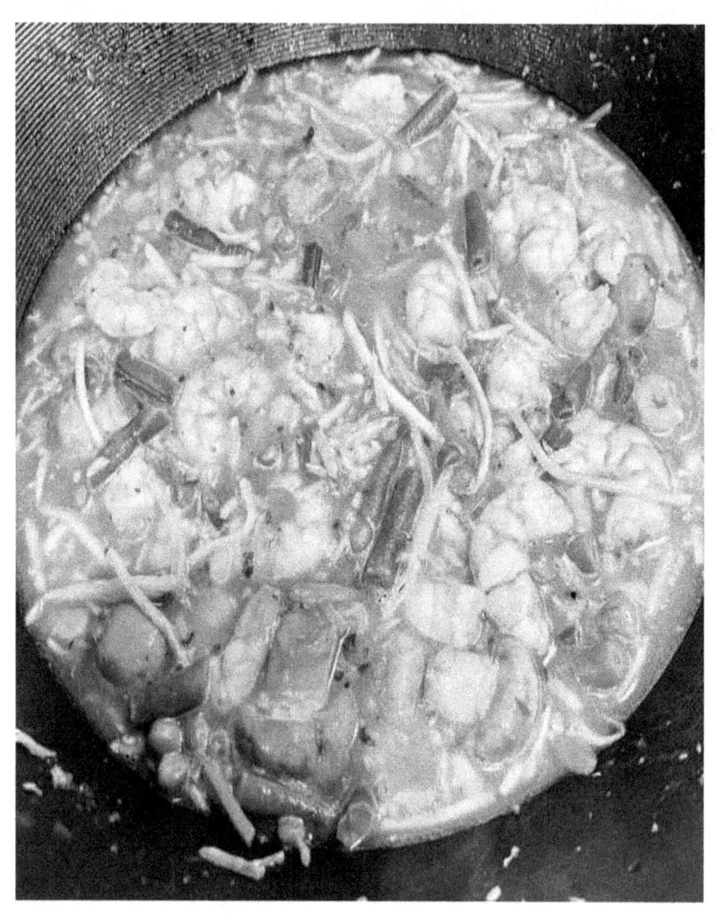

Chapter 5: Dinner Recipes

Pesto Ravioli with Tomatoes & Spinach

Ingredients:

Two 8-oz containers of cheese ravioli, either chilled or frozen

One tsp of olive oil

Grape tomatoes, one pint

One five-oz container of baby spinach

1/4 cup pesto

Instructions:

1. Bring a large pot of water to a boil. Cook ravioli as directed on the package; drain and reserve.

2. In a big, nonstick skillet, heat the oil over medium heat. Add the tomatoes and sauté for 3 to 4 minutes, or until they start to burst. After adding the spinach, simmer it for another one to two minutes, tossing it constantly, until it wilts.

3. Stir the pesto and cooked ravioli together carefully.

Filling Potatoes with Beans and Salsa

Ingredients:

Four russet potatoes, medium

1/4 cup of new salsa

1 sliced, ripe avocado

One fifteen-ounce can of washed, heated, and lightly mashed pinto beans

Chop four teaspoons of pickled jalapeños.

Instructions:

1. Use a fork to pierce potatoes all over. Microwave for about 20 minutes on Medium, rotating once or twice, or until soft. (Alternatively, bake potatoes for 45 to 1 hour at 425 degrees Fahrenheit until they are soft.) Move to a sanitized chopping board and allow it to cool somewhat.

2. To open the potato, cut lengthwise but do not cut all the way through, using a dish towel to shield your hands. To reveal the flesh, pinch the ends.

3. Some of the salsa, avocado, beans, and jalapeños should be added on the top of each potato. Warm up and serve.

White Bean & Veggie Salad

Ingredients:

Two cups mixed greens for salad

3/4 cup of your preferred vegetables, such cherry tomatoes and sliced cucumbers

One-third cup of rinsed and drained canned white beans

1/2 chopped avocado

One tsp red wine vinegar

Two tsp pure virgin olive oil

1/4 tsp kosher salt

Ground pepper freshly to taste

Instructions:

1. In a medium bowl, mix the greens, vegetables, beans, and avocado.

2. Add a drizzle of vinegar and oil, then season with pepper and salt. Transfer to a large platter after tossing to mix.

Fresh Herb Shrimp Linguini

Ingredients:

One pound of peeled and deveined medium shrimp, either fresh or frozen

Six ounces of dried linguini, packed

Grated Parmesan cheese, ¼ cup

Four minced garlic cloves

Two teaspoons of pure olive oil

1(½) tablespoons freshly chopped rosemary

Salt, ½ teaspoon

1/8 teaspoon of black pepper, ground coarsely

1 stem of rosemary

Instructions:

1. If shrimp is frozen, thaw it. Rinse the shrimp, then reserve. Cook pasta as directed on the package, leaving out the salt. In the final three minutes of cooking, add the shrimp. Once completely drained, transfer to a large spaghetti bowl.

2. Toss until well coated after adding 2 tablespoons of cheese, garlic, olive oil, chopped rosemary, salt, and black pepper.

3. If preferred, garnish with sprigs of rosemary and evenly distribute the remaining 2 tablespoons of cheese.

Sheet-Pan Caprese Pizza

Ingredients:

Freshly made, one-pound whole-wheat pizza dough
One tsp of olive oil
1/4 tsp kosher salt, separated
One-half teaspoon black pepper, split
Eight ounces of freshly sliced, thinly mozzarella cheese
Two cups of small heirloom tomatoes, cut in half or quarters
1/2 cup of fresh basil leaves, loosely packed
Half a tsp balsamic glaze

Instructions:

1. Put a 17-by-12-inch baking sheet into the oven and turn the temperature up to 450 degrees. Roll out the pizza dough onto a wide piece of parchment paper to make a rectangle that measures 15 by 10.

2. Evenly coat the dough with oil and then season with 1/4 tsp pepper and 1/2 tsp salt. Place onto a baking sheet that has been warmed. Bake for about ten minutes, or until the crust begins to color.

3. Take out of the oven; sprinkle cheese and tomatoes on top equally. Take the oven back to 450 degrees F and bake for about 2 minutes, or until the cheesc has melted.

4. Take out of the oven. Add the remaining 1/4 tsp of salt and pepper, along with the basil, and then drizzle with the glaze. Cut into six pieces.

Cauliflower Gnocchi with Asparagus and Pesto

Ingredients:
One tsp of olive oil
One 10-oz package of frozen cauliflower gnocchi.
8 ounces of trimmed asparagus spears
1/3 cup pesto basilico

Instructions:
1. In a big, nonstick skillet, heat the oil over medium heat. Add the gnocchi and simmer, turning

often, for 6 to 8 minutes, or until cooked through and golden brown.

2. In the meantime, add 1/4 inch of water to a microwave-safe plate of asparagus. Tightly cover and cook on High for approximately 2 minutes, or until crisp-tender and vibrant green. After draining, cut into 1-inch segments.

3. Toss to mix the gnocchi with the asparagus and pesto.

Creamy Mushrooms with Chicken

Ingredients:
Cutlets of chicken, 4-5 ounces
4 cups sliced mixed mushrooms, if big
1/2 cup white wine, dry
1/2 cup of thick cream
Two tablespoons of fresh parsley, cut finely.

Instructions:
1. Add 1/4 teaspoon of kosher salt and pepper to the chicken. In a big skillet, heat up one tablespoon of canola oil on medium heat. Cook for 7 to 10 minutes, rotating once, or until the chicken is browned and cooked through. Move to a platter.

2. Add the mushrooms and 1 tablespoon of oil to the pan. Cook, stirring regularly, for about 4 minutes, or until the liquid has evaporated. Turn the heat up to high, pour in the wine, and cook for

approximately 4 minutes, or until most of it evaporates.

3. Turn down the heat to medium and mix in the cream, any leftover chicken juice, and 1/4 teaspoon each of salt and pepper. Put the chicken back in the pan and flip it over to coat it with sauce. Present the chicken with the sauce on top and some parsley on top.

Skillet of Black Bean Fajitas

Ingredients:
One tsp of olive oil
One 12-oz box of chopped onions and bell peppers for fajitas
One fifteen-ounce can of drained black beans without additional salt
1/2 teaspoon salt-free seasoning mix in the Southwest
Salt, ¼ teaspoon
1/4 cup (1 ounce; optional) of finely shredded Cheddar cheese

Instructions:
1. Heat the oil in a large skillet over medium heat. Add the fajita veggies and cook for five minutes or until they are soft.

2. Add the salt, spice, and black beans and mix. Cook, stirring, for one minute or until cooked through.

3. Spoon two tablespoons of cheese, if used, over each bowl after dividing the veggies and beans amongst them.

Baked Eggs with Kale in Tomato Sauce

Ingredients:

One tablespoon of pure olive oil

Three 10-oz packets of frozen chopped kale that have been thawed, drained, and pressed dry make nine cups.

Split a ½ teaspoon of salt.

Half a teaspoon of ground pepper, split

Three cups of low-sodium tomato sauce from a can or one 25-ounce jar of low-sodium marinara sauce

Eight big eggs

Instructions:

1. Set oven temperature to 350°F.

2. In a nonstick ovenproof skillet or 10-inch cast-iron pan, heat the oil over medium heat. After adding the kale and seasoning it with 1/8 teaspoon pepper and 1/4 teaspoon salt, sauté it for 2 minutes. Add the tomato or marinara sauce, stirring, and heat through.

3. Using the back of a spoon, create 8 wells in the sauce, then delicately crack an egg into each well.

4. Add the remaining 1/4 teaspoon salt and 1/8 teaspoon pepper to the eggs to season them.

5. Place the pan in the oven and bake for about 20 minutes, or until the yolks are still soft but the whites are set.

3-Ingredient sun-dried tomatoes and chickpeas with kale

Ingredients:

One tablespoon of jarred oil and half a cup of sun-dried tomatoes packed with olive oil

One 10-oz container of finely chopped kale

1/4 cup water

One fifteen-oz can of washed, unsalted chickpeas

Instructions:

1. In a large, nonstick skillet, heat the sun-dried tomato oil over medium heat. Add the kale and simmer, stirring, for approximately 2 minutes, or until wilted and brilliant green. Reduce heat to medium-low, add water, cover, and cook for an additional three minutes.

2. Add the sun-dried tomatoes and chickpeas, and simmer, stirring, for one minute or until heated through.

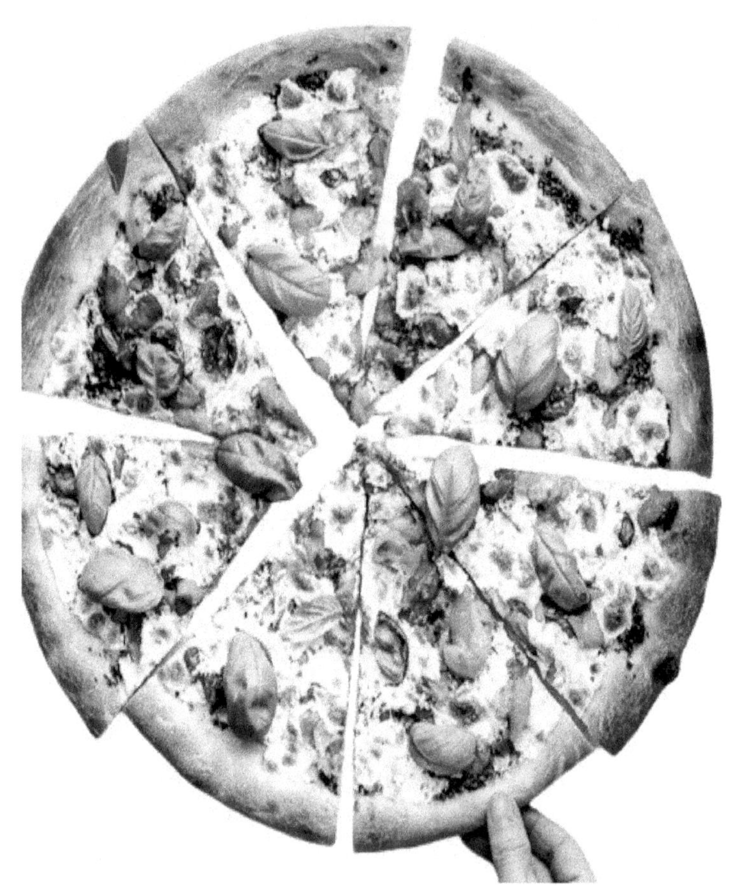

Chapter 6: Snacks Recipes

Avocado Spread

Ingredients:

One (15-oz) can of chickpeas without additional salt

One mature avocado, pitted and halved

One cup of fresh cilantro, raw

1/4 cup tahini

Extra virgin olive oil (1½ cup)

1/4 cup of lemon juice

One garlic clove

One teaspoon of cumin powder

Salt, ½ teaspoon

Instructions:

1. After draining the beans, set aside two teaspoons of the liquid. Place the conserved liquid and the chickpeas in a food processor.

2. Add the oil, lemon juice, garlic, cumin, avocado, cilantro, and tahini. Blend until very smooth. Accompany with crudités, pita chips, or vegetable chips.

Skewers of capers

Ingredients:

16 little, newly made mozzarella balls

Sixteen new basil leaves

16 miniature tomatoes

Drizzle with extra virgin olive oil

To taste, add coarse salt and freshly ground pepper.

Instructions:

Put tomatoes, mozzarella, and basil on little skewers. After adding a drizzle of oil, season with salt and pepper.

Almond-Cranberry Energy Balls

Ingredients:

1/2 cup unprocessed whole almonds

Half a cup of dried cranberries sweetened

Pitted dates, ¼ cup

1/2 cup traditional rolled oats

Twice as much tahini

Two tsp freshly squeezed lemon juice

One tablespoon of maple syrup alone

Instructions:

In a large food processor, add the almonds, cranberries, and dates. Process on High for 10 to 15 seconds, or until the ingredients are broken up into smaller bits. Stir in the tahini, maple syrup, lemon juice, and oats. Process for an additional 40 to 60 seconds, or until a thick paste develops. Using your hands, form the mixture into 25 balls, each containing approximately 1 tablespoon.

Advice:

Oats labeled "gluten-free" should be consumed by those with celiac disease or gluten sensitivity since oats can cross-contaminate with wheat and barley.

Carrot Cake Energy Bites

Ingredients;

A cup of dates with pits

1/4 cup of traditional rolled oats

Chopped pecans, ¼ cup

Half a cup chia seeds

Two medium carrots, almost 4 ounces in total, cut finely

One tsp vanilla essence

1/4 tsp finely ground cinnamon

1/2 teaspoon of ginger, ground

1/4 tsp finely ground turmeric

Salt, ¼ teaspoon

Pinch of pepper, ground

Instructions:

1. In a food processor, mix dates, oats, pecans, and chia seeds; pulse until well incorporated and diced.

2. Add the carrots, salt, pepper, turmeric, cinnamon, ginger, and vanilla; pulse until all the ingredients are thoroughly chopped and a paste starts to form.

3. Using a scant 1 Tbsp. each ball, roll the mixture.

Cauliflower Hummus

Ingredients,:
Six cups (about one pound) of cauliflower florets
One tablespoon of extra virgin olive oil + more for decoration
One huge clove of finely chopped garlic
1/4 cup tahini
Rind of one lemon
Two tsp of lemon juice
A smidgeon of kosher salt
1/2 teaspoon of cumin powder
A tsp of finely ground red pepper
Two tsp of water
Red bell pepper, chopped, for decoration
Instructions:
1. Bake at 400 degrees Fahrenheit and line a baking sheet with silicone mat or parchment paper. Toss the cauliflower with oil in a big basin. Place in a single layer on the baking sheet that has been prepared.
2. Roast for 20 to 25 minutes, or until soft and beginning to brown. Once at room temperature, let cool.
3. In a food processor, combine the cauliflower, garlic, tahini, lemon zest, lemon juice, salt, cumin, crushed red pepper, and water. Blend until well blended, stopping occasionally to scrape down the

bowl's edges. If you want a looser dip, add extra water.

4. Place in a basin. If desired, add chopped pepper and drizzle with more olive oil.

Sunflower-Apricot Granola Bars

Ingredients:
Three cups of traditional rolled oats
1 cup cereal made of crispy brown rice.
One cup of coarsely chopped, 1/4-inch dried apricots
1/2 cup toasted, unsalted pepitas
1/2 cup toasted, unsalted sunflower seeds
Salt, ¼ teaspoon
2/3 cup light corn syrup or brown rice syrup
One-fourth cup sunflower seed butter
One tsp finely ground cinnamon

Instructions:
1. Set the oven temperature to 325°F. Lay parchment paper into a 9 x 13-inch baking pan, allowing excess to hang over two edges. Apply a thin layer of cooking spray to the paper.

2. In a large bowl, mix together oats, rice cereal, apricots, pepitas, sunflower seeds, and salt.

3. In a bowl that is safe to microwave, combine cinnamon, sunflower butter, and rice syrup (or corn syrup). 30 seconds in the microwave (or 1 minute

on medium heat in a saucepan). Stir until thoroughly blended after adding to the dry ingredients. Using the back of a spatula, carefully push the mixture into the pan that has been prepared.

4. For chewier bars, bake for 20 to 25 minutes, or until the edges are just beginning to turn color but the center is still soft. For crispier bars, bake for 30 to 35 minutes, or until the edges are golden brown and the center is still slightly firm. (When heated, both will remain pliable and solidify upon cooling.)

5. Allow it cool in the pan for ten minutes, then carefully remove (it will still be soft) from the pan using the parchment paper as support. Cut into 24 bars and allow to cool fully, about 30 minutes longer, being careful not to let the bars separate. After cooling, divide into bars.

Ricotta and Yogurt Parfait

Ingredients:
3/4 cup vanilla Greek yogurt without fat
Half a cup of part-skim ricotta
Zest from ½ teaspoon lemon
Half a cup raspberries
One tablespoon of almonds, slivered
One tsp chia seeds

Instructions:

In a bowl, mix yogurt, ricotta, and zest from the lemon. Add chia seeds, almonds, and raspberries on top.

Air-Fried Kale Chips

Ingredients:
Cooking mist
Six cups of tightly packed, torn lacinato kale leaves (8 oz. bunch)
One tsp of olive oil
One and a half tsp low-sodium soy sauce
A tsp of salt
One-half tsp white sesame seeds
1/4 teaspoon of cumin powder

Instructions:

1. Cooking spray should be added to the air fryer basket.

2. In a medium bowl, toss the kale with the oil, soy sauce, and salt; thoroughly massage the leaves to coat.

3. Fill the prepared basket with the kale mixture. Sprinkle some cooking spray on the leaves. Cook for 10 to 12 minutes at 375 degrees Fahrenheit, shaking the basket and stirring the leaves every 3 to 4 minutes, or until crispy. Take out of the basket and immediately toss with the cumin and sesame seeds.

Peach and Pistachio Toast

Ingredients:

One tsp part-skim ricotta cheese

One tsp honey, separated

1/2 tsp cinnamon

One toasted piece of 100% whole-wheat bread

1/2 sliced medium peach

1/4 cup finely chopped pistachios

Instructions:

1. In a small dish, mix together ricotta, cinnamon, and ½ teaspoon honey.

2. Toast is spread with the ricotta mixture, then peach and pistachios are added. Pour in the last of the 1/2 teaspoon honey.

Garlic and Rosemary Pecans

Ingredients:

One big egg white

Three teaspoons of finely chopped dried rosemary

Two tsp of salt with garlic

3-cups pecans

Instructions:

1. Turn the oven on to 250°F.

2. In a larger bowl, whisk together egg white, garlic salt, and rosemary. Toss in the pecans to coat. Arrange evenly on a large baking sheet with a rim.

Bake for approximately 45 minutes, stirring every 15 minutes, or until dry. Allow it cool entirely, about 30 minutes, before storing.

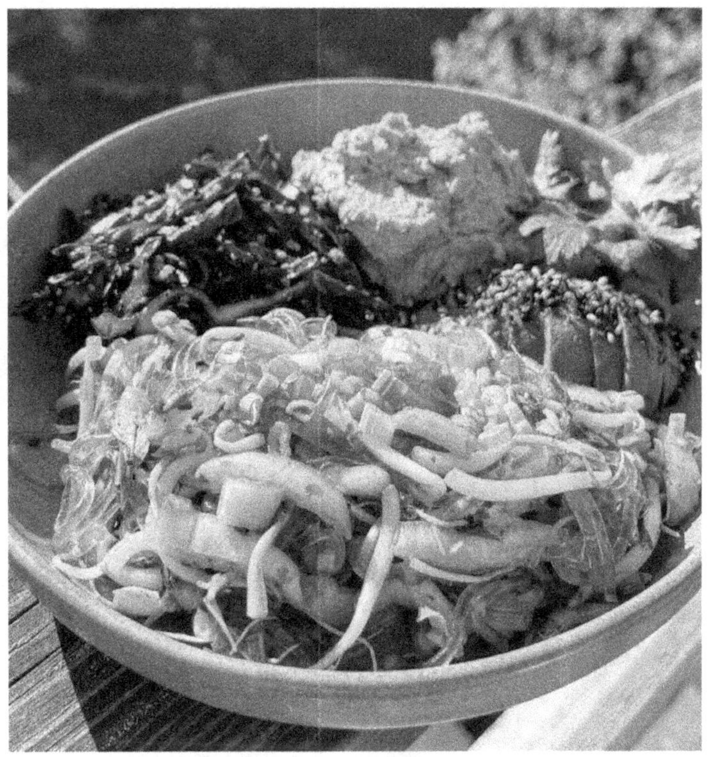

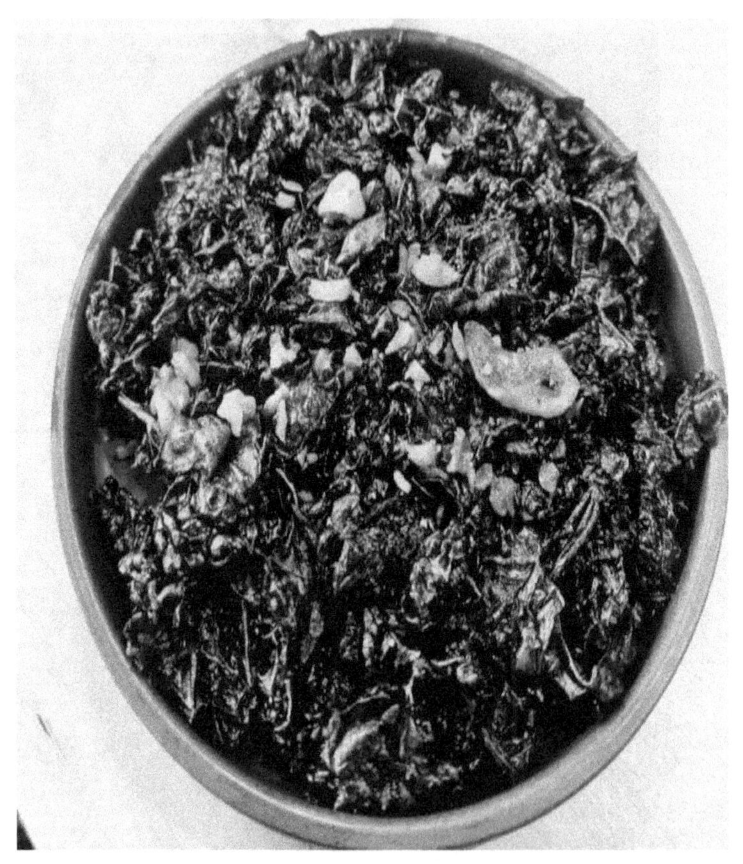

Chapter 7: Dessert Recipes

Spiced Roasted Apples

Ingredients:

One pack contains 1/2 to ½ cup of brown sugar

1/2 tsp powdered cardamom or cinnamon

Six cups of fresh fruit, such as grapes, sliced pears, or berries

Three tablespoons of butter, melted

Optional: ricotta cheese, yogurt, or oatmeal

Crunchy Oats (optional)

Instructions:

1. Preheat the oven to 450°F. In a separate dish, mix the brown sugar and cardamom.

2. Place parchment paper inside a 15 × 10 inch sheet pan. Divide the fruit evenly in the prepared pan. Sprinkle with powdered sugar and brush with butter.

3. Fruit should be baked uncovered for 10 to 15 minutes, or until it begins to color and soften. Permit to cool somewhat. If preferred, top with Crispy Oats and serve alongside oats, yogurt, or ricotta. Makes 4 servings.

Using Twisted Oats:

1. Preheat the oven to 350°F. Combine 1 cup of quick-cooking or regular-cooking oats with 3 tablespoons of packed brown sugar and melted butter. Evenly spread into the baking pan and bake at 350° for 15 minutes, stirring once.

2. Remove and let cool in the pan. Transfer to a storage container. Cover and keep at room temperature for up to 3 days, or freeze for up to 1 month.

Lemon cake and olive oil

Ingredients:

A solitary spoonful of melted butter
1/2 cup of granulated sugar
1/2 cup almonds, slivered and roasted
Two cups of all-purpose flour
Four teaspoons of finely grated lemon peel
1/3 tsp of baking powder
1/2 teaspoon salt
A half-cup of juice from lemons
Three eggs, gently beaten
One cup of buttermilk
Extra virgin olive oil, half a cup
One-half tsp almond extract
Two cups of seasonal, freshly sliced fruit*
Twist-up of granulated sugar

Sugar powder (optional)

Instructions:

1. Turn the oven on to 375°F. Lightly mist a 9-inch cake pan or a 10-inch cast iron skillet with the butter; put aside.

2. Place the almonds and 1/2 cup of granulated sugar in a food processor. After the mixture is finely blended, cover and pulse repeatedly on and off. Move to a large bowl. Add the baking powder, salt, flour, and lemon peel and stir until combined. In the center of the flour mixture, make a well and set it aside.

3. Whisk together eggs, buttermilk, almond essence, olive oil, and three tablespoons of lemon juice in a medium-sized bowl. Add everything at once to flour mixture, stirring just until combined. Evenly distribute batter in a skillet that has been prepared.

4. In case you're using a cake pan, bake it for 30 minutes instead of 25 minutes, or until a wooden toothpick inserted in the center comes out clean. Allow the cake to cool in the pan on a wire rack for minimum of fifteen minutes. Meanwhile, in a medium-sized dish, combine the fruit, the remaining 3 tablespoons lemon juice, and the 2 tablespoons granulated sugar.

5. If desired, dust the cake with powdered sugar. The fruit combination can be served warm or room temperature.

Mint Greek Frozen Yogurt

Ingredients:
Basic, low-fat (2%) Greek yogurt in three cups
One sugar cup
1½ cups freshly squeezed lemon juice
Two tsp flour
One teaspoon salt
Two tsp finely chopped fresh mint
Instructions:
1. In a medium-sized bowl, combine the yogurt, sugar, lemon juice, vanilla, and salt. Whisk until smooth.
2. Freeze the yogurt mixture in an ice cream maker with a 1 1/2 to 2 quart capacity, as directed by the manufacturer.
3. Add mint and stir. Transfer to an airtight container and freeze for two to four hours before serving. Allow to remain at room temperature for five to fifteen minutes before serving.

Triple Chocolate Tiramisu

Ingredients:
Split into two 3-oz packets of ladyfingers

A quarter-cup of robust espresso or coffee

One 8-oz container of mascarpone cheese

A single cup of rich cream

1/4 cup powdered sugar

One teaspoon vanilla

1/3 cup of cocoa liquor

Grated white chocolate, one ounce, for making bars or squares

A single ounce of chocolate, grated and bittersweet

Sugar-free cocoa powder

Coating coffee beans with chopped chocolate is optional.

Instructions:

1. Line the bottom of an 8 x 8 x 2 inch baking pan with a few ladyfingers, cutting to fit if necessary. Drizzle half of the espresso over the ladyfingers and set aside.

2. In a medium-sized mixing basin, beat together the mascarpone cheese, whipping cream, powdered sugar, and vanilla with an electric mixer until stiff peaks form. Add the chocolate liqueur and beat just until blended.

3. Evenly distribute half of the mascarpone mixture over the ladyfingers using a spoon. Over the mascarpone mixture, sprinkle bittersweet and white chocolate. Add another layer of ladyfingers on top (keep any extras for a different purpose). Add the

remaining mascarpone cheese mixture and espresso on top.

4. For six to twenty-four hours, cover and refrigerate. Dust the dessert with chocolate powder. Add chocolate beans for decoration if you'd like.

5. Yields twelve squares.

Strawberry and Sweet Ricotta Parfait

Ingredients:

One pound of freshly cut, quartered or halved strawberries

One tsp sugar

1 tablespoon of freshly chopped mint

One carton of fifteen ounces of part-skim ricotta cheese

3 teaspoons of light agave nectar.

Half a teaspoon vanilla

Half a teaspoon of lemon peel, roughly chopped

Fresh mint

Instructions:

1. In a medium-sized bowl, combine strawberries, sugar, and 1 tablespoon finely chopped mint; toss gently to combine. Let stand for about ten minutes, or until berries start to release their juices and become softer.

2. In another medium bowl, combine the ricotta, vanilla, agave nectar, and lemon peel. Use an electric mixer on low medium speed for two minutes.

3. Before assembling, fill each of the six parfait glasses with one tablespoon of the ricotta mixture. Each glass should have a generous spoonful of the strawberry mixture spread over the ricotta mixture.

4. Repeat layering with remaining ricotta and strawberry mixes. If preferred, additional sprigs of fresh mint can be used to top. You may either serve it immediately or keep it in the fridge for up to four hours.

Tart with Honey-Lavender Flavor

Ingredients:
One cup of flour, for everything
1/4 cup powdered sugar
1/4 teaspoon salt
1/2 cup of unsalted butter melted
1/4 cup of honey
Three tsp of food-grade dried lavender buds
One spoonful of gelatin, plain
Four large oeufs.
3/4 cup of granulated sugar
4 lemons, 1 tsp zest and 1/2 cup juice
Two tablespoons of unsalted butter, cut into slices

Whipped cream

Caramelized Lemons

Instructions:

1. In a larger bowl, stir together flour, powdered sugar, and 1/4 tsp salt. Stir the dough until it comes together after adding melted butter. Press dough evenly into the bottom and up the sides of a 9-inch round or 14-by-4-inch rectangle tart pan with a removable bottom. Chill the crust for at least 20 minutes, or until it solidifies.

2. Preheat the oven to 350°F. Prick the whole bottom of the crust with a fork. Pie weights or dry beans can be used to fill the crust that has been lined with parchment paper or foil. a bake of 20 minutes. After removing the foil and pie weights, bake for a further 10 to 15 minutes, or until the crust is golden. To cool, place on a wire rack.

3. Place honey and lavender buds in a small pot to produce lavender honey. On medium heat, bring the honey to a simmer. Stirring occasionally, simmer over medium-low heat for fifteen minutes. Turn off the heat and let it sit for fifteen minutes. Pour the honey through a fine-mesh filter to extract the lavender, then throw away the strainer. Store the honey.

4. In a small dish, sprinkle the gelatin over four tablespoons of cold water and set aside.

In a medium saucepan, thoroughly whisk together eggs, granulated sugar, and lemon zest. Pour in the lemon juice and mix. Cook over medium heat, whisking often, for 6 to 8 minutes, or until thick and creamy. (Lemon curd leaves a streak on the back of a spoon; rub your finger over it to see it.)

4. Remove the curd from the heat and stir in the melted butter. Stir in the gelatin until well combined. (The heat will cause the gelatin to melt.) Pour curd over the cold crust. Refrigerate the tart for four hours or until it solidifies completely.

5. Top the tart with whipped cream and candied lemons. Add a drizzle of lavender honey. has 8 servings in it.

Chocolate Almond Butter Fruit Dip

Ingredients:

One cup of plain Greek yogurt

1/2 cup almond butter

1/3 cup chocolate-hazelnut spread

One-third teaspoon honey

One teaspoon vanilla

Fresh fruit in slices, such as apples, bananas, pears, apricots, and/or bananas

Instructions:

In a medium-sized dish, combine the first five ingredients (through vanilla). For a smoother, lighter dip, place in a food processor or blender, cover, and pulse until smooth. Serve with fruit.

Ginger-Turmeric Barley Pudding

Ingredients:
Three full glasses of milk
A half-cup of uncooked pearl barley
1/2 cup of honey or sugar crystals
Grated and peeled 2-inch piece of fresh ginger (two packed teaspoons)
A single cinnamon stick
1/2 teaspoon of coarsely chopped nutmeg
A pinch of Kosher salt
Half of a vanilla bean
Two yolks from eggs
Half a teaspoon of powdered turmeric
Dense brown sugar, halved
One and a half-inch piece of raw ginger, peeled and diced (about half a teaspoon)
1/3 cup chopped Medjool dates with pits
1/4 teaspoon salt
Instructions:
To make pudding;

1. In a large saucepan, mix together milk, barley, granulated sugar, nutmeg, cinnamon stick, 2 tsp. fresh ginger, and a little sprinkle of salt. Remove the seeds by cutting a vanilla bean in half lengthwise. Add seeds and pod to pan. Reduce the heat after bringing it to a simmer over medium-high heat. For thirty minutes, simmer gently covered, stirring periodically.

2. In a small dish, whisk together egg yolks and turmeric. Stir in approximately 1 cup of the heated barley mixture gradually. After adding the egg mixture to the pan, simmer it gently for one minute, or until it thickens and reaches 195°F on a thermometer. Turn off the heat and let it cool somewhat. Take out and throw away the vanilla pod and cinnamon stick.

To make Date-Ginger Syrup

1. In the meanwhile, regarding date-ginger syrup: In a small saucepan, simmer the brown sugar, 1/4 cup water, and 1/2 tsp ginger over medium-high heat.

2. Cover and simmer until the syrup reduces to half a cup, about 3 minutes. Remove from the heat and stir in the dates, another 1/4 tsp salt, and two to three milligrams of black pepper.

3. If necessary, add one to two teaspoons of water to get a pourable consistency. Use immediately or refrigerate until needed. Pour date-ginger syrup

over pudding and serve warm or chilled. Makes 4 servings.

Pears poached in cider in a slow cooker Four medium-ripe, firm pears

Ingredients:
2 cups of apple cider
One teaspoon of honey
One 3-inch stick of cinnamon
One-third cup of crystallized ginger, coarsely chopped
Two green cardamom pods were crushed to extract the seeds.
1/2 cup vanilla-flavored Greek yogurt
Two teaspoons finely chopped pistachios
Four medium-ripe, firm pears
2 cups of apple cider
One teaspoon of honey
One 3-inch stick of cinnamon
One-third cup of crystallized ginger, coarsely chopped
Two green cardamom pods were crushed to extract the seeds.
1/2 cup vanilla-flavored Greek yogurt
Two teaspoons finely chopped pistachios

1. In a 4- to 6-quart electric or stovetop pressure cooker, stir the following 5 ingredients (up to cardamom) until the honey melts. Arrange the pears in the cooker. Put the lid lock in place.

2. Cook in an electric cooker under high pressure for 5 minutes. In a stovetop cooker, raise the pressure to a medium-high level and then reduce the heat just enough to maintain the pressure without going overboard. Simmer for 5 minutes.

3. Discontinue the heat. Quickly release the pressure in both cookers. Lift the lid gently. Using a slotted spoon, transfer the pears to dessert plates, leaving the cider mixture on the stove.

4. On an electric cooker, use the sauté setting and steadily boil, uncovered, until the mixture turns syrupy, 12 to 15 minutes. Use the stovetop cooker directly in the saucepan to cook. Recool a little.

5. After straining through a fine-mesh strainer, discard the spices. Spoon the cider syrup over the pears. Add yogurt and pistachios as garnish.

To slow-cook on high for two hours:

1. In a 3 1/2 or 4-quart slow cooker, combine the first five ingredients (up to the cardamom) and stir until the honey dissolves.

2. Arrange the pears in the cooker. After two hours of cooking on high with a cover, the pears ought to

be just tender. With a slotted spoon, transfer the pears to dessert plates. Transfer the simmering liquid into a compact saucepan and bring it to a rolling boil.

3. Boil gently, uncovered, for 12 to 15 minutes, or until syrupy. Recool a little. After straining through a fine-mesh strainer, discard the spices. Spoon the cider syrup over the pears. Add yogurt and pistachios as garnish.

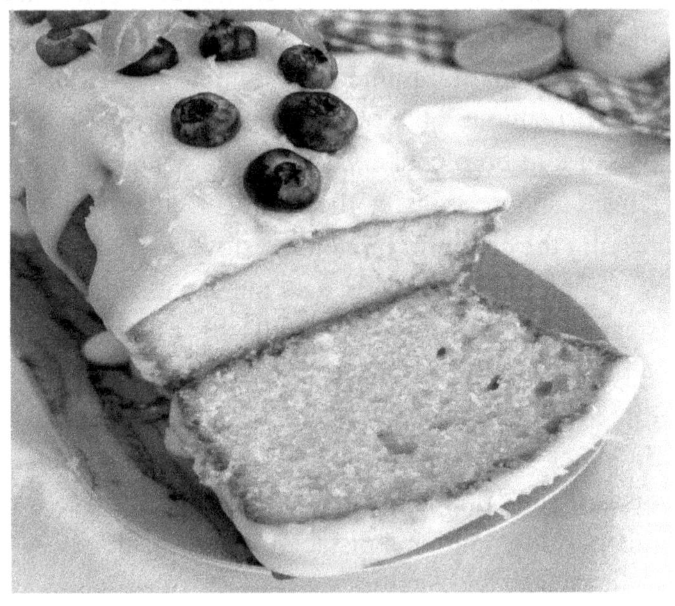

Chapter 8: 10-Page Meal Planner Bonus

Weekly Meal Plan

	Breakfast	Lunch	Dinner
Monday	Fast-cooking cereals	Mustard Potato Salad	Pasta with vegetables
Tuesday	Southwest-style Quesadilla	Avocado spread	Sheet-pan caprese pizza
Wednesday	Egg Salad Toast with avocado	Skewers of capers	Cauliflower Gnocchi with asparagus & pesto
Thursday	Margarita Egg Pancake	Almond-cranberry energy balls	Creamy mushrooms with chicken
Friday	Mustard Chickpea	Filling spinach & Chickpea stew	Skillet of black bean fajitas
Saturday	Chickpea & Kale Toast	Filling Minestrone	Baked eggs with kale in tomato sauce
Sunday	Tabouli bowl	Strawberry and sweet ricotta parfait	3-ingredient sun-dried tomatoes & chickpeas with kale

Weekly Meal Plan

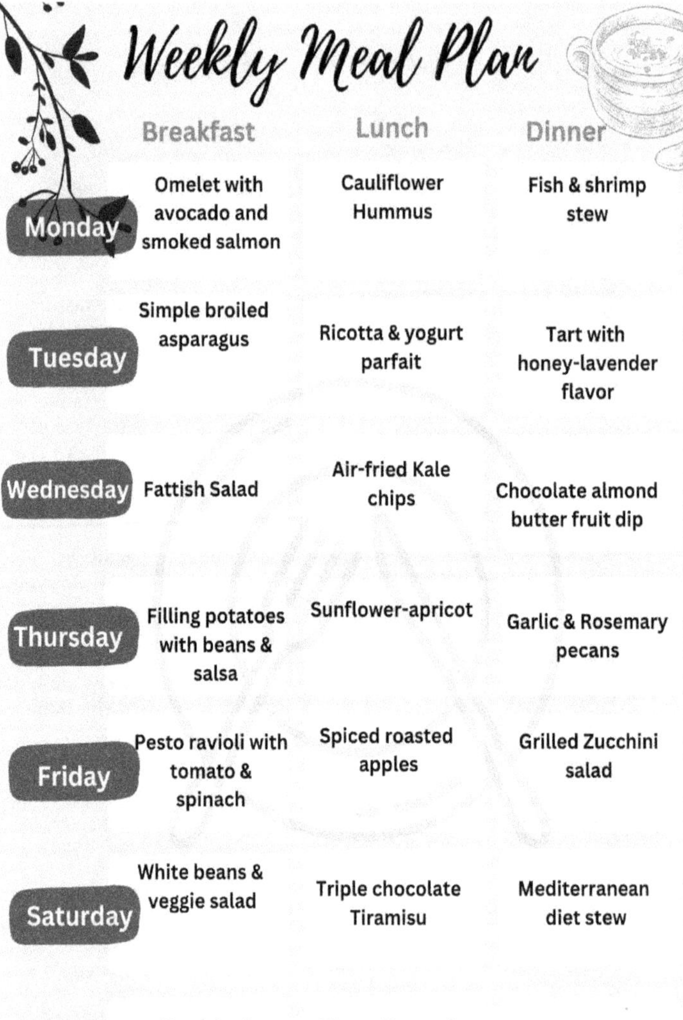

	Breakfast	Lunch	Dinner
Monday	Omelet with avocado and smoked salmon	Cauliflower Hummus	Fish & shrimp stew
Tuesday	Simple broiled asparagus	Ricotta & yogurt parfait	Tart with honey-lavender flavor
Wednesday	Fattish Salad	Air-fried Kale chips	Chocolate almond butter fruit dip
Thursday	Filling potatoes with beans & salsa	Sunflower-apricot	Garlic & Rosemary pecans
Friday	Pesto ravioli with tomato & spinach	Spiced roasted apples	Grilled Zucchini salad
Saturday	White beans & veggie salad	Triple chocolate Tiramisu	Mediterranean diet stew
Sunday	Fresh herb shrimp linguini	Ginger-Turmeric barley pudding	Peach & Pistachio toast

Weekly Meal Plan

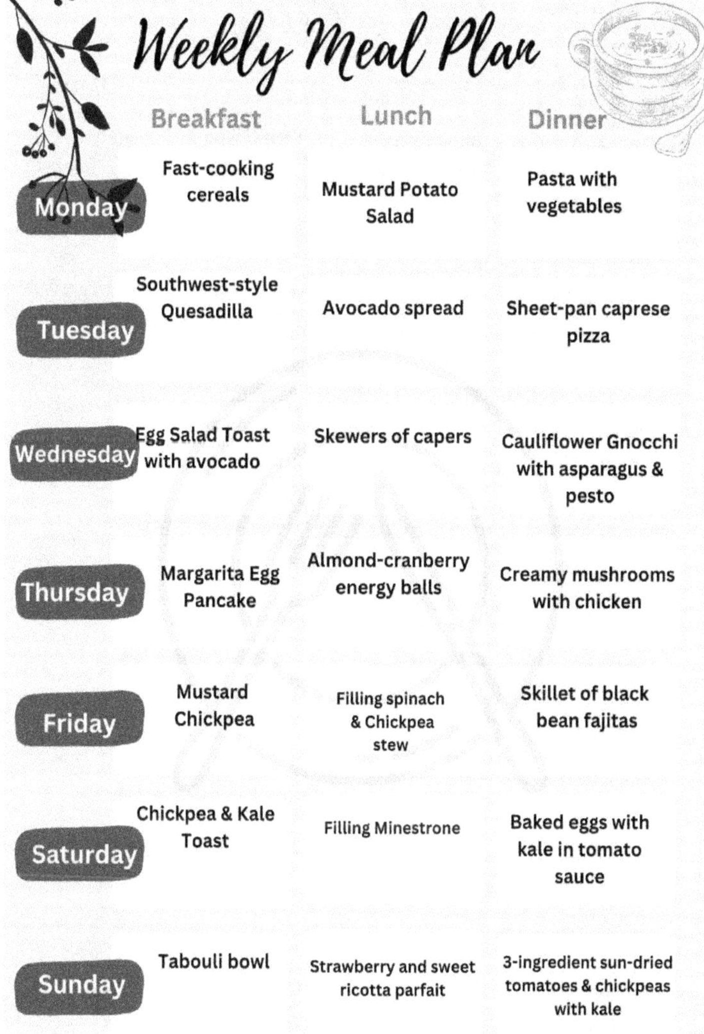

	Breakfast	Lunch	Dinner
Monday	Fast-cooking cereals	Mustard Potato Salad	Pasta with vegetables
Tuesday	Southwest-style Quesadilla	Avocado spread	Sheet-pan caprese pizza
Wednesday	Egg Salad Toast with avocado	Skewers of capers	Cauliflower Gnocchi with asparagus & pesto
Thursday	Margarita Egg Pancake	Almond-cranberry energy balls	Creamy mushrooms with chicken
Friday	Mustard Chickpea	Filling spinach & Chickpea stew	Skillet of black bean fajitas
Saturday	Chickpea & Kale Toast	Filling Minestrone	Baked eggs with kale in tomato sauce
Sunday	Tabouli bowl	Strawberry and sweet ricotta parfait	3-ingredient sun-dried tomatoes & chickpeas with kale

Weekly Meal Plan

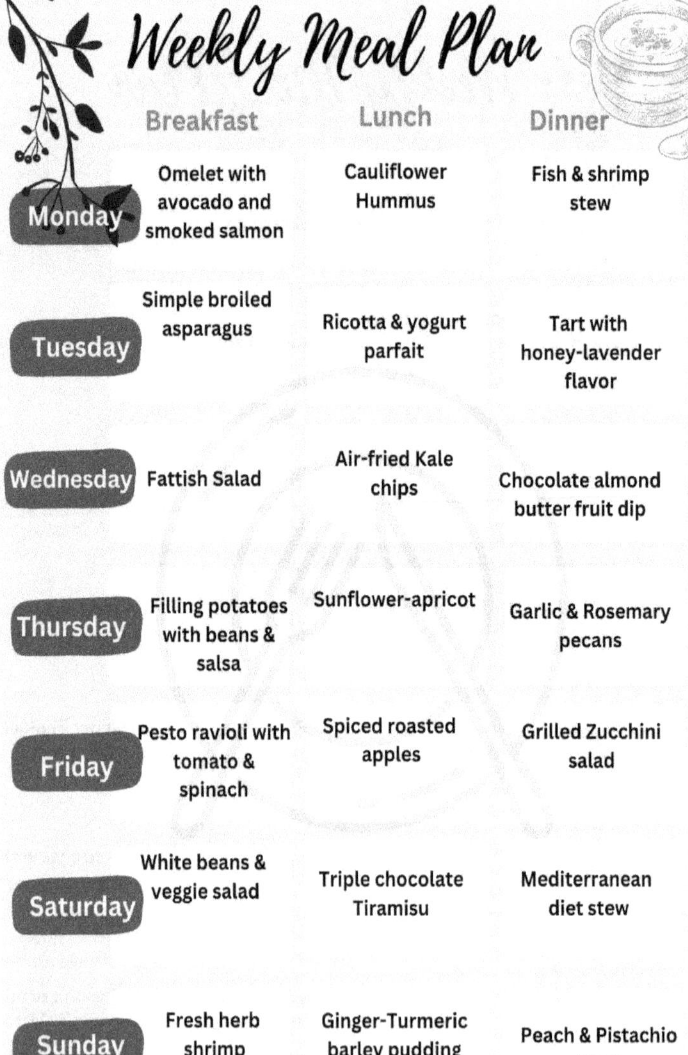

	Breakfast	Lunch	Dinner
Monday	Omelet with avocado and smoked salmon	Cauliflower Hummus	Fish & shrimp stew
Tuesday	Simple broiled asparagus	Ricotta & yogurt parfait	Tart with honey-lavender flavor
Wednesday	Fattish Salad	Air-fried Kale chips	Chocolate almond butter fruit dip
Thursday	Filling potatoes with beans & salsa	Sunflower-apricot	Garlic & Rosemary pecans
Friday	Pesto ravioli with tomato & spinach	Spiced roasted apples	Grilled Zucchini salad
Saturday	White beans & veggie salad	Triple chocolate Tiramisu	Mediterranean diet stew
Sunday	Fresh herb shrimp linguini	Ginger-Turmeric barley pudding	Peach & Pistachio toast

Weekly Meal Plan

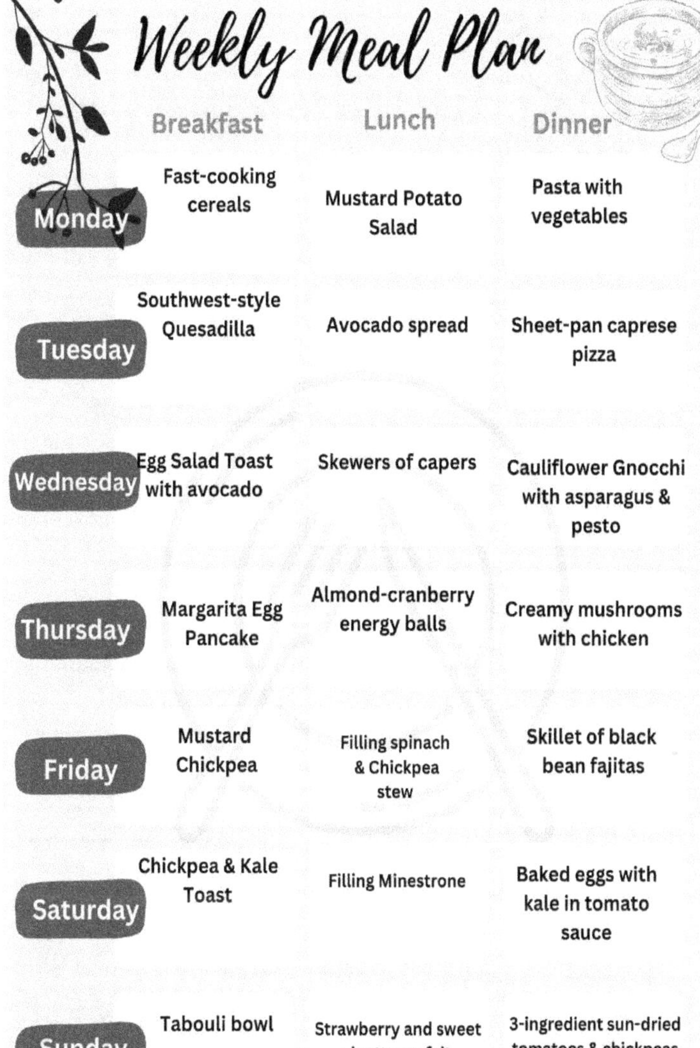

	Breakfast	Lunch	Dinner
Monday	Fast-cooking cereals	Mustard Potato Salad	Pasta with vegetables
Tuesday	Southwest-style Quesadilla	Avocado spread	Sheet-pan caprese pizza
Wednesday	Egg Salad Toast with avocado	Skewers of capers	Cauliflower Gnocchi with asparagus & pesto
Thursday	Margarita Egg Pancake	Almond-cranberry energy balls	Creamy mushrooms with chicken
Friday	Mustard Chickpea	Filling spinach & Chickpea stew	Skillet of black bean fajitas
Saturday	Chickpea & Kale Toast	Filling Minestrone	Baked eggs with kale in tomato sauce
Sunday	Tabouli bowl	Strawberry and sweet ricotta parfait	3-ingredient sun-dried tomatoes & chickpeas with kale

Weekly Meal Planner

WEEK ___________   DATE ___________

MONDAY

TUESDAY

WEDNESDAY

THURSDAY

FRIDAY

SATURDAY

SUNDAY

NOTE

TO EAT IS A NECESSITY, BUT TO EAT INTELLIGENTLY IS AN ART.

Weekly Meal Planner

WEEK ___________________   DATE ___________________

MONDAY

SATURDAY

TUESDAY

SUNDAY

WEDNESDAY

NOTE

THURSDAY

FRIDAY

TO EAT IS A NECESSITY, BUT TO EAT INTELLIGENTLY IS AN ART.

Weekly Meal Planner

WEEK ______________________   DATE ______________________

MONDAY

SATURDAY

TUESDAY

SUNDAY

WEDNESDAY

THURSDAY

NOTE

FRIDAY

TO EAT IS A NECESSITY, BUT TO EAT INTELLIGENTLY IS AN ART.

Weekly Meal Planner

WEEK ___________________

DATE ___________________

MONDAY

TUESDAY

WEDNESDAY

THURSDAY

FRIDAY

SATURDAY

SUNDAY

NOTE

____

____

____

____

____

TO EAT IS A NECESSITY, BUT TO EAT INTELLIGENTLY IS AN ART.

Weekly Meal Planner

WEEK _______________   DATE _______________

MONDAY

TUESDAY

WEDNESDAY

THURSDAY

FRIDAY

SATURDAY

SUNDAY

NOTE

TO EAT IS A NECESSITY, BUT TO EAT INTELLIGENTLY IS AN ART.

Conclusion

Compared to other adults, those who eat a Mediterranean diet live longer and experience fewer chronic illnesses.

Plant-based foods including fruits, vegetables, whole grains, legumes, and nuts are emphasized in the Mediterranean diet. It employs herbs and spices rather than salt to flavor food and swaps out butter for healthy fats like canola and olive oil. Fish should be served twice a week and red meat no more than a couple times per month.

A Mediterranean diet may also reduce the incidence of type 2 diabetes and its complications, according to additional research. There are several explanations on why this can be the case.

It has been demonstrated that a 58% reduction in the incidence of type 2 diabetes can be achieved by increasing physical activity, losing weight, and consuming less saturated fat and more dietary fiber.

Numerous of these nutritional features are present in the Mediterranean diet, such as high antioxidant levels, moderate intake of saturated fat, and high fiber content. A correlation has also been shown between a Mediterranean-style diet and a decrease in the incidence of diabetes complications including retinopathy, according to a cross-sectional study conducted in Melbourne.

Even while the Mediterranean diet may lower your chance of developing some chronic illnesses, if losing weight is one of your objectives, you still need to pay attention to portion sizes. Consuming a diet high in fats and oils might result in an excess of kilojoules and weight gain. Therefore, it's critical to maintain an active lifestyle, eat a range of nutrient-dense meals from the five food categories, and consume food in accordance with your energy demands in order to promote general health and lower the risk of issues.

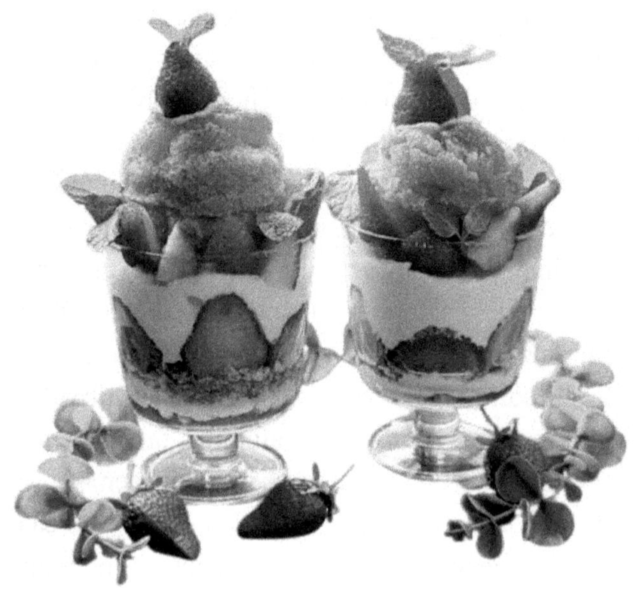